THE BLUNT NUTRITIONIST

12 Weeks to Weight Loss

(With Tough Love and Brutal Honesty)

AMIE HORNAMAN,
NUTRITIONIST AND FUNCTIONAL MEDICINE PRACTITIONER

Medical Disclaimer: The Blunt Nutritionist/Amie Hornaman is providing this book and its contents on an "as is" basis and makes no representations or warranties of any kind with respect to this book or its contents.

You understand that the suggestions and guidance in this book is provided without a health examination and without prior discussion of your health condition. You understand that in no way will The Blunt Nutritionist/Amie Hornaman provide medical advice without a one on one consultation.

The information in this book is not intended as medical advice, medical nutrition therapy or individualized nutrition counseling/coaching. This book and its author does not claim to cure, prevent, diagnose, or treat any nutrition-related disease or health condition. Always consult a qualified healthcare professional before changing your diet or medications or beginning any exercise routine.

The nutrition information provided in this book is provided for personal and informational purposes only. You should always consult with a competent, fully licensed medical professional when making any decisions regarding your health. The author of this book will use reasonable efforts to include up-to-date and accurate information but make no representations, warranties, or assurances as to the accuracy, currency, or completeness of the information provided. The authors of this site shall not be liable for any damages or injury resulting from your access to this book and/or it's information, or from your reliance upon any information provided in this book.

You understand that these services are not intended as a substitute for consultation with a licensed healthcare practitioner, such as your physician. Before you begin any weight loss or fitness program, or change your nutritional regimen, you will consult your physician or other licensed healthcare practitioner to ensure that you are in good health and that these services will not harm you.

You understand that the information and content of these services should not be used to diagnose a health problem or disease, or to determine any health-related treatment program, including weight loss, diet, or exercise.

You understand that there are risks associated with the use of these services. Use of these services implies that you assume all risks, known and unknown, inherent to exercise, workout programs, nutrition programs, and physical changes and/or injuries which may result from the use of these services.

Copyright © 2018 **Amie Hornaman**

All rights reserved. No part of this book nor its products or publications may be reproduced, transmitted, transcribed, stored in a retrieval system, or translated into any language, in any form, by any means, without the written permission of the author. All information and supporting resources are developed solely for your personal use and may not be reproduced for publication or for the personal or commercial use of others without express permission from the book's author. www.amiehornaman.com

ISBN-13: 978-1721617630
ISBN-10: 1721617639

Photo Creds: Jennifer White, Acacia Studios www.iloveacacia.com

Testimonials

I would like to share my experience with Amie as my nutritional coach because it has been such an amazing one! After trying so many diet plans in the past that ultimately failed, I was left frustrated with my weight and concerned for my overall health. I later suffered an injury that made working out impossible, and I was afraid losing weight would be an even more difficult task. I decided one day to have a consult with Amie and give her personalized program a try, and in weeks I saw big results! I was shocked since I was not able to move around much at all. She tailored a nutrition program to me that made losing the unwanted pounds so easy. Throughout the process there definitely have been challenging times when I came close to giving up, and this is where Amie was so radically different from other coaches and programs I attempted: when typically in the past I'd throw in the towel, now with her guidance and encouraging words, I was not dropping the ball! This is by far my favorite part of this experience! Amie always knows what to say and more importantly how to say it. It's like she knows exactly what you need to hear to stay on track and it made an enormous difference! Now, 6 months and 50 pounds later, I cannot recommend her program enough! It isn't really a "program" more like life changing guidance to help you focus on health rather than size, which as a healthcare professional I truly appreciate! Good luck and talk to Amie if you want to finally make that change! - Lauren

I was desperate when I finally found Amie. I am a 56 year old, 50 pound overweight woman. I have tried almost all of the diet plans out there, and I continued to gain 5 pounds every year. I felt like I was dying, high cholesterol, borderline high blood pressure. I was so out of breath walking the dog. Amie was my last chance. I couldn't believe how great I felt within one week of working with Amie. It's not really a DIET! She customizes a food plan just for you. If you have cravings for certain foods she makes suggestions that you can live with. Who loses weight during the holidays! Well, I do! I am down 12 pounds already. And I feel satisfied. She worked with my doctor and convinced them to order more blood tests that established to them that I did indeed have an autoimmune thyroid condition. Thanks to Amie I am now getting the proper medication and proper food choices. It's not always about getting a bikini body, sometimes it's just about feeling like you are finally living! - Patty C.

Amie came into my life during a tough and trying time. I always thought I had PCOS, but doctors never showed any signs of wanting to confirm my fears. After finally getting pregnant and enduring a rough pregnancy and delivery, I pushed hard enough and got tested. While it was nice to finally have confirmation, I didn't know where to go from there. Doctors put me on some basic meds and tried to get me to go on diets that will do more harm than good to those that have this condition. All of the appointments and contradicting instructions I was given was not helping me in any shape, way, or form. My weight was out of control, and I finally reached my breaking point. I felt like crap all of the time, and that's not ideal when you have an

infant to chase after. That's when I found Amie. She is someone that I can relate to on many levels. Amie is a wealth of knowledge and a great coach. Even with a great coach though, I still fell off track. My husband lost his job, my grandmother passed away a month later, and I underwent shoulder surgery a month after that. If I thought I hit a low before, it was nothing like what I was going through then. With the exception of my husband and son, I shut everyone out, and that included Amie. After several months, I finally started to pick myself up and reached back out to her. She welcomed me back with open arms, and it was the farthest thing from what I was expecting. It was nice to know that someone understood and reminded me that I am only human. I am proud to call her a friend. Focusing on my health again has helped pick me up out of the funk, and currently, I am down 12 pounds in 6 weeks. I still have quite a bit to go, but with Amie's guidance and encouragement, I am optimistic to reach this goal by the end of the year.
- Katelyn

Amie cares! You'll receive a personalized plan, lots of helpful tips, & one on one support. If you're serious about changing bad habits then take this next simple step to a healthy life! - Hayley S.

I have been working with Amie for less than a year and couldn't be happier with my results. She is extremely knowledgeable and dedicated to fitness and nutrition. With a warm yet no nonsense attitude she pushes me beyond my own limits. Not only is she my nutritionist and massage therapist, I feel she has become a friend. Not only have I become stronger I have incredible energy for my yoga practice. Thank you Amie, I am loving my new muscles!
- Charla

Working with Amie Hornaman as a personal trainer has been life changing for me. She has made it possible for me to not only enjoy my workouts, but also look forward to them. She is a well-rounded trainer that offers personal training and professional nutritional advice that is realistic for my very busy lifestyle. I have lost 4 pants sizes, 10lbs and gained the knowledge and confidence I need to make this a lifestyle change for my family and myself. Thank you Amie for your help and support you are amazing!!! - Rachel

Thanks Amie Hornaman! It has been one of the best experiences in my life! I've gone through years of physical therapy and never got the results I've got working out with you! The time spent in the gym was well worth it! I completed 4 months of personal training. I lost over 20 pounds, I'm stronger and able to do so much more physically! I'm so grateful for the patience she took with me! For those who may not think they will achieve results because they are too old, I proved that wrong! Being 59 years old and in bad shape before, I have come a long way with Amie's help and encouragement. I got great results! Thanks again Amie. - Marcia

INTRODUCTION

There is a very good reason my clients call me the *"Blunt Nutritionist,"* I'm not going to tell you what you want to hear, I'm gong to tell you what you NEED to hear. And, sometimes you won't like it.

I could make you promises that sound SUPER enticing to make you buy this book, but where would that get either of us? You won't feel any better, and my reputation is toast. So that won't work. I think its better to be brutally honest with you and sprinkle that with tough love. I promise if you do what I tell you to do and make some changes to your routine your whole world will be changed! But it won't be a quick fix. This workbook will take you on a journey to better health, weight loss and a better belly… but it won't always be easy or comfortable.

"Better health" is a very vague term so let's quickly explain what that means. It means you'll be less bloated after eating, and you'll have better digestion when you eat. "Better health" means the best version of you at a better weight if you have a few to lose, whether it's those last 5 lbs or 50 lbs. And, finally, "better health" means you'll have more energy throughout the day instead of wanting to take a nap at 2 pm, which is pretty exciting! As I write this it's 2:23 pm, and this used to be the time in the day where my eyes would close and the couch in my office started looking VERY inviting! Those days have long passed, and I'm happy to say I can not only get through the day with energy, but I also pay attention to what's going on around me   which is always a bonus in business. I have finally reached a point where I can have a brownie without putting on 5 lbs in a day, but I also don't crave brownies like I used to. That's what I want for you!

My goal for you in this journey to better health is to walk you step by step through important questions about your health, discussing how you feel along the way. Together we will be figuring out what symptoms you struggle with and take you week by week through gradual changes that equal long term results.

I promise to always be honest and upfront with you as to what to expect.

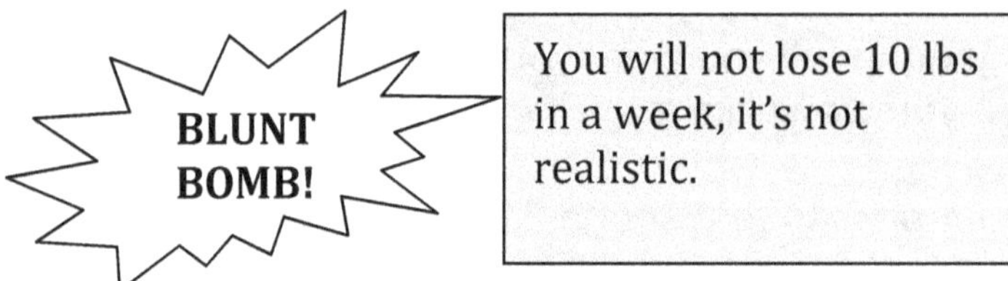

Honestly, you probably won't even notice the scale move until week 4. But that's okay if we are making lasting changes. If we break through your health barriers and make permanent change, who cares how long it takes?! So let's move on to week 1…

Week 1: Honesty

Goals: Record 3 days of EVERYTHING you eat and drink. It can be any 3 days of the week. Try to pick one weekend day and 2 days during the week. Do not try to eat like you just joined Weight Watchers because you have to write your food down. Journaling your food and being honest lets us figure out your cravings, patterns and habits. Be honest with yourself. It's amazing how this will open your eyes to what ACTUALLY goes into your mouth.

> ***Nutrition Rule #167:***
> You will eventually eat any food that is in your house if you like it. You will see how true that is when you write down every bite that goes into your mouth.

Questions to answer: This week we want to explore the foods you crave and the patterns to your blood sugar.

1. Do you crave sweet or salty foods?

____
____
____

2. Does your appetite increase at night?

____
____
____

3. What time of day do you get the most hungry?

____
____
____

4. Do you experience extreme hunger or "sugar lows" at all through the day (moodiness, light headedness, dizziness, extreme hunger)?

____

____

____

Journal the times of day when you are hungry. What do you tend to crave... and ultimately eat... when you are hungry? If you answered yes to question 4, document the details. Did you go too long without eating? What did you eat through the day? When you felt moody and hungry, what did you end up eating?

What to Expect Week 1: Realistically, you are just beginning. Don't be hard on yourself if you have garbage food in your journal. Our goal is to explore and get real. Let's see what your cravings are so we can work together to find replacement foods for them.

Day 1: What did I eat today? What time(s) of the day did I eat?

____

____

____

____

____

____

Day 2: What did I eat today? What time(s) of the day did I eat?

____

____

____

____

____

____

Day 3: What did I eat today? What time(s) of the day did I eat?

____

____

____

____

____

____

Week 2: Blood Sugar

Goals: Record 3 days of EVERYTHING you eat and drink. It can be any 3 days of the week. Try to pick one weekend day and 2 days during the week. This week we are going to work at replacing the foods you crave and the foods you reach for when you experience low blood sugar.

In Week 1 you identified foods that you crave. Look back at what you wrote down and list those foods here that contain high amounts of sugar, white flour or come in a package:

____

____

____

____

____

This week whenever you crave those foods listed above replace them where you can with foods from this list:

86% dark chocolate
Blue corn tortilla chips
Sweet potato chips
Terra chips
Hummus and vegetables
Almond flour chocolate chip cookies (see fastpaleo.com for some amazing recipes)
Gluten free almond flour brownies
3 gluten free cookies (store bought)
½ cup So Delicious coconut milk ice cream
Arctic Zero Ice cream (you can eat the whole pint!)
RX Bars
Coconut flakes
¼ cup nuts

We are also going to start addressing your digestion AND your blood sugar this week so just trust me and do this: take 1 capful of Braggs Organic apple cider vinegar with the "mother" in 8 oz of water (warm or cold, lemon or no lemon) and drink this first thing in the morning, with or without food.   We've all heard how apple cider vinegar is good for everything and amazingly enough IT IS. This is a simple, INEXPENSIVE way to start your day and get digestion on track. Week 3 we will be addressing your digestion anyways so why not start now. Apple cider vinegar is also known for its blood sugar balancing properties.

> ***Nutrition Rule #29:*** If it's simple and cheap just try it.

We will talk more about insulin resistance and type 2 diabetes in a later chapter, but for now we are looking at your erratic blood sugar symptoms. As discussed earlier if you feel blood sugar highs and lows or crave bread, pretzels and sugary foods later in the day then your blood sugar is on a roller coaster ride. If you feel moody and light headed when you don't eat…then your blood sugar is on a roller coater ride.

The good news is there is something you can do about it! Changing your eating is one piece. The second piece is one of the best supplements to come out in years. It's called Berberine and studies show it works as well as the type 2 diabetic/insulin resistant drug, metformin, without the side effects. It has strong antioxidant as well as lipid protective qualities (meaning it helps with those cholesterol numbers!) and is amazing at reducing sugar cravings.

My patients ultimately end up losing weight because their blood sugar comes back into balance and they crave less sugar. So as we are going through making these changes to your nutrition…and remember these are LASTING changes….you may want to think about adding in Berberine to your arsenal. Of course, make sure you speak with your doctor first about adding a supplement especially if you have an underlying health issue. But, here is the link to my favorite brand and favorite company. They are a family owned company and this is what I use with my patients to get results:
https://onenutrition.ehealthpro.com/products/berberine-synergy

What to expect in Week 2: Slightly-improved digestion. No weight loss yet!(just being honest with you). Hang in there with me a few more weeks to see the scale move or your clothes fit better.

Nutrition rule #254: what you do this week will show up next week. What you did last week shows up this week.

Day 1: What did I eat today? What time(s) of the day did I eat?

____
____
____
____
____
____

Day 2: What did I eat today? What time(s) of the day did I eat?

____
____
____
____
____
____

Day 3: What did I eat today? What time(s) of the day did I eat?

____
____
____
____
____
____

Week 3: Digestion

Goals: We are still recording 3 days worth of eating. Get used to this because we will do it the whole way through. Make note of how many times you successfully replaced your sugary, starchy foods with some of the replacement foods from Week 2:

____

____

____

This week we will be discussing digestion. We started improving your digestion by adding in apple cider vinegar and replacing some foods. Let's answer some questions about digestion now to see what we are dealing with down in that GI tract:

Do you have any of the following? Check the symptoms that apply to you:

- Peptic/Duodenal Ulcer
- Poor Appetite
- Excessive Appetite
- Gallstones
- Gallbladder Pain
- Nervous Stomach
- Full Feeling After Small Meal
- Indigestion
- Heartburn
- Acid Reflux
- Hiatal Hernia
- Nausea
- Vomiting
- Vomiting Blood
- Abdominal Pains/Cramps
- Gas

☐ Diarrhea

☐ Constipation

☐ Changes in Bowels

☐ Rectal Bleeding

☐ Tarry Stools

☐ Rectal Itching

☐ Use Laxatives

☐ Bloating

☐ Belch Frequently

☐ Anal Itching

☐ Anal Fissures

☐ Bloody Stools

☐ Undigested Food in Stools

That's a lot of symptoms I know, but all relevant to the digestive process. Have you heard that immunity starts in the gut? And weight loss starts in the gut? And disease starts in the gut? It actually does and there is science to back it.

I would encourage you along your wellness journey to do some research on the gut and how it impacts your ability to lose weight. But what you need to know this week is how to immediately improve digestion and feel less bloated. When we are bloated we feel uncomfortable in our clothes no matter what our weight may be. So this week we are going to remove dairy. Yes, I just said dairy. Stay with me…

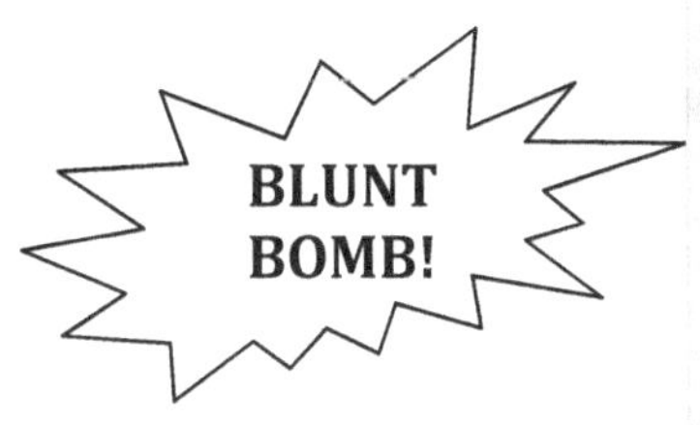

No one can digest dairy. Not you. Not me. We simply don't have the enzymes to digest dairy. We are the only species to drink another species milk. And everyone is lactose intolerant. If someone tells you they're not lactose intolerant ask them what happens when they eat ice cream. Gassy much? Bloated like you're 5 months pregnant? THAT is not being able to digest dairy.

So how can we replace dairy? How can I possibly ask you to remove milk from your cereal? What are you going to put on pizza and eat with your wine if you can't have cheeeeeeesssse (I hear you whining. You're reaching for that block of cheddar right now because you want to get it all in before you have to give it up.) Giving up cheese actually isn't that hard. First, try almond milk, coconut milk, cashew milk or rice milk. All of those milk choices taste great in cereal! Leave the soy milk on the shelves as it wreaks havoc with your hormones and thyroid.

Next…a hidden secret…goat cheddar cheese. We can digest goat milk way better than cow's milk. I don't recommend goat milk. But I HIGHLY recommend goat cheddar! Shreds like a really fresh mozzarella.

So let's journal this in your 3 days! Try these replacements and see how you do. Write it down!

If your belly went down, and your jeans button… document it! You'll want to look back and remind yourself what worked if you fall off the wagon later.

What to expect: Flatter bellies. Happier bellies. MAYBE your clothes fit a little better but don't even think about getting on the scale yet.

If you want Biggest Loser results then quit your job and workout 8 hours a day. That is the only way to lose 10 lbs a week. And by the way that weight loss is not going to last (see the "where are they now" episodes). Real weight loss, lasting weight loss, takes time.

> ***Nutrition Rule #54: Patience is a virtue.*** It just is. So when you're busting your butt doing all the right things, and you don't see the scale move yet, remember rule #54.

Day 1: What did I eat today? What time(s) of the day did I eat?

____
____
____
____
____
____

Day 2: What did I eat today? What time(s) of the day did I eat?

____
____
____
____
____
____

Day 3: What did I eat today? What time(s) of the day did I eat?

____
____
____
____
____
____

Week 4: Sleep

Goals: Continue with the 3-day food journaling! We need to keep tracking and making changes. But this week we are ALSO going to track your sleep. Believe it or not sleep plays a HUGE role in hormone balance, blood sugar control and weight loss. If you're not sleeping, you won't lose weight. Plain and simple. So let's see how you are doing…

Is your energy low through the day?

○ Yes ○ No

Do you have trouble getting to sleep?

○ Yes ○ No

Does your energy increase at night?

○ Yes ○ No

Do you have trouble staying asleep?

○ Yes ○ No

How many hours a night do you sleep? _______________________

What do you eat before bed? _________________________________

That should give you some insight as to whether or not you are sleeping well…although you probably already knew that. The food before bed questions tie in with blood sugar control. If you eat foods that are processed, high in sugar, high in starchy carbohydrates such as pretzels/pizza/beer, then you will have a spike in blood sugar before bed and a low blood sugar in the middle of the night. This is often a cause of people waking in the middle of the night and is definitely a cause of extreme hunger in the morning. Document, be honest, and make some changes. Refer back to Week 2 for ideas of replacement foods.

You may have heard this all before, but I'm going to repeat it for you…get away from blue light before bed! Phones, computers, ipads and TV. Blue light reduces our body's ability to produce melatonin, the hormone required to relax us and get us ready for sleep. Our brain essentially thinks its still daylight when we stare at our phones and computers in the evening, and we never receive that signal that its time for our bodies to shut down. Filter what you can with an orange light screen. Most phones now have the option to lower the light automatically at a certain time of night. There are apps that offer an orange light screen. There are glasses on Amazon that are blue light filtering so you can still watch TV up until you hit the hay. We now know how important sleep is to overall health, so why not go the extra mile?

Do you simply work yourself to death and go to bed too late? Do you not get enough sleep? If the answer is yes and yes, are you willing to change that? It's going to require you actually NOT work up until 10 pm. If you aren't willing to change that nasty habit then I'm going to be brutally honest with you since that's the theme of the book, you will never be healthy and you most likely won't lose weight. Yes, you might make more money because you are the classic workaholic, but you won't be alive long enough to enjoy it. **Truth.**

> *Nutrition rule #89:*
> People who have
> trouble getting to sleep
> and staying asleep
> increased their risk of
> a FATAL heart attack
> by 18-27 percent,
> regardless of age,
> weight, smoking and
> exercise habits.

These statistics were taken from 15 different studies of over 160,000 people. Craziness! NOW do I have your attention on how important sleep is to our bodies? Let's shoot for 6-8 hours each night this week, shall we?

What to expect: With all of the changes we have made in the last 4 weeks your digestion should be greatly improved, your belly bloat down and your clothes fitting better. You may even start to see a pound or 2 come off the scale. Refer back to the "what to expect" section of Week 3 if you are getting frustrated.

Day 1: What did I eat today? What time(s) of the day did I eat?

____
____
____
____
____
____

HOW MANY HOURS DID I SLEEP? ____________________

Day 2: What did I eat today? What time(s) of the day did I eat?

____
____
____
____
____
____

HOW MANY HOURS DID I SLEEP? ____________________

Day 3: What did I eat today? What time(s) of the day did I eat?

____
____
____
____
____
____

HOW MANY HOURS DID I SLEEP? ____________________

Day 4: HOW MANY HOURS DID I SLEEP? ________________

Day 5: HOW MANY HOURS DID I SLEEP? ________________

Day 6: HOW MANY HOURS DID I SLEEP? ________________

Day 7: HOW MANY HOURS DID I SLEEP? ________________

Week 5: Stress

Goals: Still document 3 days of eating! You should have a good handle on your sleep patterns so you can stop documenting your sleep. Hopefully you've made some changes to your sleep to get a minimum of 6 hours. This week's goal is to address stress. Now…let's be clear. Everyone has stress and it's hard to escape, reduce or minimize. Some situations such as death and divorce you just have to get through. Ongoing work stress of "I hate my job," you either change or learn how to deal with your choice of situation. Almost everyone has money stress (except Oprah). And, the stress of having kids…well, kudos to you for taking that on. You give everything up for your kids, and they only make you gray and fat. Not much you can do about that stress. Drink wine and wait until the day you can give them the best birthday present ever…suitcases for their 18th birthday! So you see where I'm going? We have to manage how we DEAL with stress, because it's not going away.

Questions:

Do you feel like you can't handle stress very well?

____

____

Do you feel overly emotional on a daily basis?

____

____

Do you lack motivation to do daily activities?

____

____

Does it feel like you get a "second wind" at night?

____

____

Do you have a hard time getting up in the morning?

____

____

That should give you an insight into how you are handling stress. The energy increasing at night and energy low in the morning might indicate that your cortisol levels are unbalanced. Cortisol is our stress hormone that is released by the adrenal glands when we are stressed out. It can be released in a burst such as running from an attacker, or it can be released in long waves such as hating your job. When cortisol is released in an ongoing fashion it tends to store fat in the abdomen. That's not fun and doesn't serve us well in our health journey. So what can we do about it? Manage it. Alter your perception of stress.

> ***Nutrition rule #5:***
> ***Pick your battles.***
> Extra stress is not
> worth extra fat on your
> belly.

Example: You hate your job because Suzy Q makes your life miserable every day, but you have to put up with her because she is one position above you and isn't leaving anytime soon. You can either, A. Quit your job, Or B. Give a nickname for Suzy in your head, but DON'T say it out loud. Make it one that makes you giggle a bit inside every time you see her. Ask yourself if Ms. Suzy is worth ruining your day as you bring your bad mood home to the family.

What to expect: Clothes fitting better, more energy, better sleep and a few more pounds lost on the scale. Oh, and definitely less water retention and bloating.

Day 1: What did I eat today? What time(s) of the day did I eat?

____

____

____

____

____

____

Day 2: What did I eat today? What time(s) of the day did I eat?

____
____
____
____
____
____

Day 3: What did I eat today? What time(s) of the day did I eat?

____
____
____
____
____
____

Week 6: Movement and Exercise

Goals: Yes, you're still tracking 3 days of food choices. Now, we're going to start tracking movement and exercise. What counts as movement? Walking, yoga, hot yoga, exercise videos or classes, crossfit, running, rowing, jazzercise, dancing, zumba, step class, any cardio equipment, weight training etc.

ANYTHING that puts your body into action counts as movement. For right now, your goal is 2 times a week, and if you get in more... BONUS for the WIN! But, we're shooting for twice a week. That's really not too much to ask and anyone can do it. Always remember we are shooting for long-term lifestyle changes, not just temporary results.

How long should you be "moving"? Minimum 20 minutes. If you're doing high intensity exercise like Cross-fit you can do 15 minutes and be done. If you're walking for your movement, then 20-30 minutes is optimal.

What to expect this week: Greater regularity. Also enjoy more mental clarity and less brain fog. You should be seeing the scale move by now. If it hasn't moved yet, you may need to call me for a one-on-one consultation because you might have a medical condition holding you back from losing weight. Yes, you can call the author! See the services section at the end of the book.

Day 1: What did I eat today? What time(s) of the day did I eat?

____

____

____

____

____

____

MOVEMENT CHOICES: ______________________________

Day 2: What did I eat today? What time(s) of the day did I eat?

____

____

____

____

____

____

MOVEMENT CHOICES: _______________________________________

Day 3: What did I eat today? What time(s) of the day did I eat?

____

____

____

____

____

____

BONUS DAY! MOVEMENT CHOICES:_______________________________

Week 7: Do you REALLY want to change?

Goals: To keep plugging away. And MOVE three times a week!

Compare your first week of food journaling to this week. How many foods are different? Better? If you've made less than 5 changes we may need to dig a bit deeper as to the why.

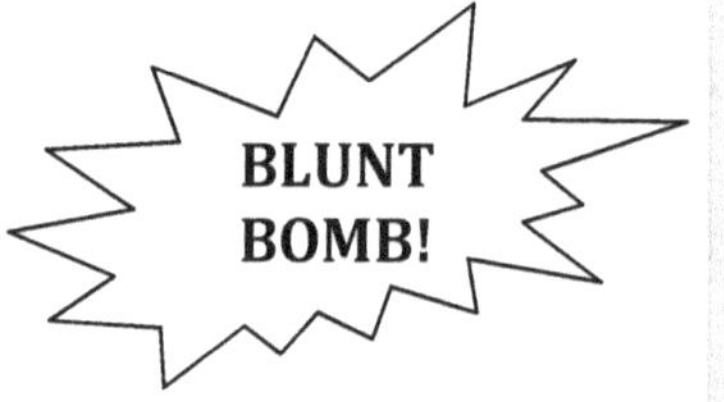

If you are on Week 7 and have made LESS than 5 total changes in food, sleep habits, moving your body and addressing stress, then maybe you really don't WANT to change!

You have to want it. I have patients who ask me, "what can you do to help my husband, wife, sister, friend (insert friend or family member here) get healthy and lose weight?" I tell them I can't do anything if they don't want to change, so it always has to start there.

So take a moment, dig deep and ask yourself…are you ready to change? What is holding you back? What kind of motivation do you need? Do you need more accountability? More support? Maybe you should consider working this program with a friend? Only you can answer those questions. Write your answer below so you can see it in front of you. Once you see it in writing you'll be more likely to do something about it:

____
____
____
____
____
____

And, if you ARE making some radical life altering changes then good for you! Keep tracking.

Day 1: What did I eat today? What time(s) of the day did I eat?

____

____

____

____

____

____

MOVEMENT CHOICES: ____________________________

Day 2: What did I eat today? What time(s) of the day did I eat?

____

____

____

____

____

____

MOVEMENT CHOICES: ____________________________

Day 3: What did I eat today? What time(s) of the day did I eat?

____

____

____

____

____

____

MOVEMENT CHOICES: ____________________________

Week 8: Is your thyroid making you fat?

Goals: Keep tracking your food and exercise. Keep looking at stress and sleep as these can get off track easily and quickly.

This week we are gong to be looking at your thyroid:

Questions:

Have you gained weight that you can't take off?

____

Do you put on weight easily?

____

Have you not lost weight yet on this program?

____

Are your nail beds wavy, have ridges or lines in them or break easily?

____

Do you retain water easily?

____

Are you sensitive to cold or heat?

____

Do you experience randomized anxiety?

____

Is your energy low through the day?

____

Are you often constipated?

____

Is your hair thinning or falling out?

____

If you answered "yes" to 5 or more questions you MAY have a thyroid problem. The thyroid is the master of your metabolism. It gives you the ability to lose weight, have energy, not loose your hair, be in a good mood and sleep well. If it is off you won't even want to get out of bed in the morning. MOST of the time it is difficult to get your thyroid under control without some professional intervention. We need to do testing; proper, thorough testing. You need someone to look at that testing to see if your numbers are OPTIMAL, not just normal. You need medication or a darn good supplement that works like a medication if your thyroid is slow.

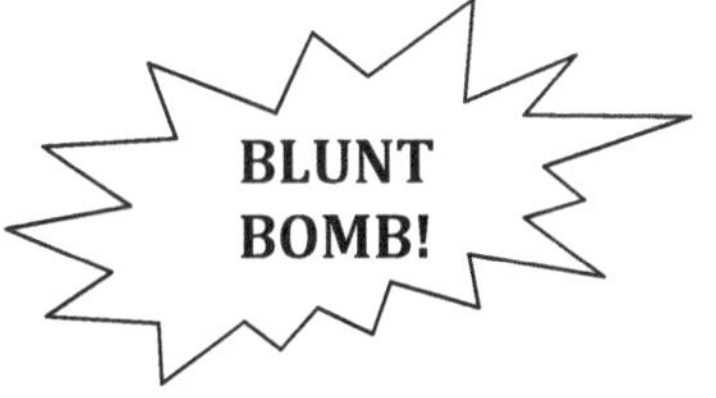

If someone tells you that you can heal your thyroid with food...RUN. You can help it to work better and reduce inflammation, but you cannot FIX a clinically low thyroid with food.

I could write a book within a book right here on the thyroid. It looks like I will be writing you another book so you can learn about the master controller of your body, but for now let's just start to get an idea of how yours is working and what you can do. Answer the questions above, and if you suspect you have a low thyroid EMAIL ME, CALL ME, CONTACT ME. Tell me what other book you have read where the author tells you to call her?? Take advantage of professional advice and don't struggle on your own. I fix patients in a matter of weeks. It can be done, and I guarantee you're not the toughest case I've seen.

What to expect: weight loss as long as you don't have a thyroid problem. Regularity as long as you don't have a thyroid problem. Better energy as long as you don't have a thyroid problem.

Day 1: What did I eat today? What time(s) of the day did I eat?

____

____

____

____

____

MOVEMENT CHOICES: _______________________________

Day 2: What did I eat today? What time(s) of the day did I eat?

____

____

____

____

____

MOVEMENT CHOICES: _______________________________

Day 3: What did I eat today? What time(s) of the day did I eat?

____

____

____

____

____

MOVEMENT CHOICES: _______________________________

Week 9: Is insulin making you fat?

Goals: keep tracking your food and exercise 3 days a week. Our goal for this week is to figure out if anything else is going on underneath the surface that we need to address to get you to your goals.

Ever hear of insulin resistance? Does type 2 diabetes run in your family? Have you ever been diagnosed with PCOS (Poly Cystic Ovarian Syndrome)? Insulin resistance is the precursor to diabetes. It's the stage where your cells start becoming resistant to insulin and we don't want that. When insulin can't get into the cells it "bounces back" in to the bloodstream and sets you up for fat storage. In addition to not being healthy for your body overall, if you're trying to lose weight, having insulin resistance is not going to be beneficial to the cause. It not only prevents you from losing weight even when you're really trying, but it also allows your body to lay down fat at a rapid pace. Ever feel like you just look at a brownie sideways and gain weight?

Questions to ask yourself:

Do you have type 2 diabetes in your family?

____

Do you gain weight when trying to lose weight?

____

Have you ever been diagnosed with PCOS?

____

Do you feel like your blood sugar is on a roller coaster?

____

If you answered "yes" to one or more questions, then it might be time to get some blood-work done. Just the basics here. I'm talking about a CMP maybe an A1C. Don't know what those are? No problem, your doc will.

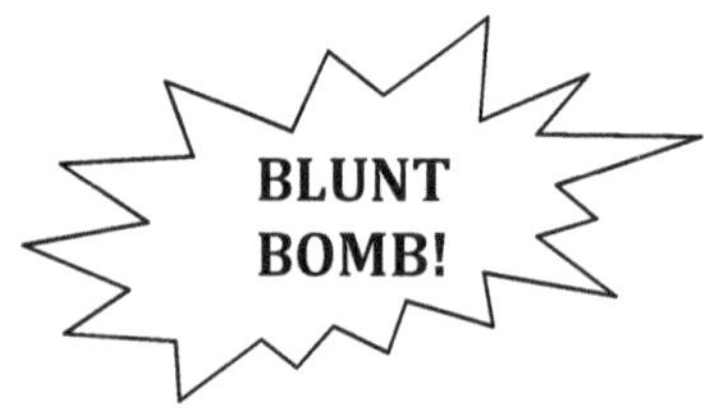

If you ask your doctor to run a test on you because you suspect something is wrong, and he/she says no...it's time to get a new doctor.

If some numbers come back askew, but you are told you are "normal," then reach out to me! We will get into optimal numbers in a different book, but just to give you a little tidbit: anything above a 90 for glucose indicates insulin resistance. I once consulted with a wise doc ahead of his time specializing in diabetes who stated that every number above an 85 increases a person's risk for type 2 diabetes by 3%. So once you hit the functional medicine optimal range you're already at a 15% increased risk. Once you hit the standard lab value ranges that are still considered to be "non diabetic" your risk has increased by 45%.

What to expect: weight loss on the scale as long as you don't have undiagnosed insulin resistance. You should be seeing/feeling improvement in everything by now if you have been making the changes you should be.

Day 1: What did I eat today? What time(s) of the day did I eat?

____
____
____
____
____
____

MOVEMENT CHOICES: ____________________________

Day 2: What did I eat today? What time(s) of the day did I eat?

____
____
____
____
____
____

MOVEMENT CHOICES: _________________________________

Day 3: What did I eat today? What time(s) of the day did I eat?

____
____
____
____
____
____

MOVEMENT CHOICES: _________________________________

Week 10: The environmental enemies

Not everyone will have to complete Week 10. Some of you are rock-stars when it comes to what you put in your body, on your body and what you use to clean your house. Read through the list for this week, and if you're already there then mad props to you. If you're like the rest of us and can use some changes, woohoo! Then read on. Regardless of where you are in your journey, everyone will be completing the basic weekly goals (even if you're getting sick of writing down your food).

Goals: Keep tracking 3 days of food because this is the time-frame where you start letting a little bit more slip in. At the same time, continue tracking your exercise, because this is where you start taking days off and let lazy slip in. And, finally…let's look at environmental factors and start chipping away at that.

Environmental factors: Things that go **on** your body (body wash, lotion, makeup, perfume), things that go **in** your body (toothpaste, mouthwash, coffee going through paper filters or Keurig), things you put your food in (Tupperware, water bottles), and things you clean your house with (glass, kitchen, toilets).

Make a list of everything you use so we can cross reference the ingredients. Maybe take a photo of the back of your products that list ingredients so we can easily go through and check them with the "dirty dozen" list below…

____

____

____

____

____

There is an 80/20 rule when it comes to changing environmental factors…80% you can control, 20% you can't control, and in that 20% there are items you will choose not to change. Hair dye…I will always get my hair colored, that's part of my 20%. Have a favorite concealer that's not on the approved list? Maybe that's part of your 20%.

But where we **can** make changes, let's make them.

Here are the top ingredients to avoid when it comes to your makeup:

- Fragrance
- Parabens
- Triclosan
- Formaldehyde-Releasing Preservatives
- Sodium Laureth Sulfate
- Petroleum distillates
- Phthalates
- PEG compounds
- Benzophenone
- Homosalate
- Siloxanes

I may be missing some, but this will get you started. If you're interested in WHY to avoid them, look each ingredient up and read about it. Ever watch one of those documentaries where they show a slaughterhouse and after you're done watching you swear never to eat a steak again? That's kind of what you'll experience. Once you know what these ingredients do to your metabolism, cells, hormones, etc., you will forever avoid them like the plague.

After you swap out the bad and get into a new routine with the good. You won't go back. Your new, chemical -free lifestyle will stick. Over time you will feel better and "cleaner" so to speak. This is a long-term goal. Exposure to chemicals have long-lasting effects on the body. Time to make another life change…

Day 1: What did I eat today? What time(s) of the day did I eat?

____
____
____
____
____
____

MOVEMENT CHOICES: _______________________________

Day 2: What did I eat today? What time(s) of the day did I eat?

____
____
____
____
____
____

MOVEMENT CHOICES: _______________________________

Day 3: What did I eat today? What time(s) of the day did I eat?

____
____
____
____
____
____

MOVEMENT CHOICES: _______________________________

Week 11: What do we still need to work on?

Let's review. Remember you can ALWAYS go back and redo any week that you need. No one cares if you make this a 13 or 14-week journey instead of 12. Do what you need to do.

Do you still need blood work done? Revisit Weeks 8 and 9. For goodness sake, ask me for help if you believe you have a thyroid condition or insulin resistance.

Is your digestion better or do you need to revisit Week 3?

____

Are you still getting sugar highs and lows and still craving sweets in mid-afternoon? Go back and repeat Week 2.

____

Did you get off track with your sleep? Go back to Week 4 and repeat.

____

Did you start letting little "bites of "sneak in? As in…a bite of ice cream, just a bite of your kid's mac n' cheese, a bite of your husband's fries? It's easy to self-sabotage at this point especially if you have seen the scale move. Document any foods you have let sneak through. Are you rationalizing that just a "bite of" is okay here and there? And BE HONEST with yourself! Journal 3 days of food, but highlight where the "bites of" are coming in to sidetrack your diet.

Movement-wise we are going to end this journey with a bang! Your goal for this week: 5 days of movement/exercise. If you haven't tried 5 days yet or ANY days yet, this is the week to try! It doesn't mean that every week will be a 5-day exercise week, but this is your crowning celebration week…so go for it. You might get sore and achy, but that will be your body thanking you for moving. You can treat yourself to 5 days of hot yoga. What a great way to detox! Or walk 5 days in the woods. Walk 5 days on the beach. Just move! Simple, yet gratifying goal.

Day 1: What did I eat today? What time(s) of the day did I eat?

____
____
____
____
____
____

MOVEMENT CHOICES: ______________________________________

Day 2: What did I eat today? What time(s) of the day did I eat?

____
____
____
____
____
____

MOVEMENT CHOICES: ______________________________________

Day 3: What did I eat today? What time(s) of the day did I eat?

____
____
____
____
____
____

MOVEMENT CHOICES: ______________________________________

Day 4 MOVEMENT CHOICES: _______________________________

Day 5 MOVEMENT CHOICES: _______________________________

Week 12: Putting it all together and moving forward.

This is the last week you are going to journal your food. You should have a pretty good grasp on your patterns by now, and after last week you should be able to tie everything together to see where you may need to focus a bit more. Take a good hard look at it at the end of the week and go back through it all with a fine-toothed comb. I think you can be honest with yourself on a daily basis now and either say, "Holy cow, I made it through a picnic without eating 10 cookies" or "holy cow, I let my cravings get the best of me today!" I've been honest with you for the past 12 weeks so it's time for you to be honest with yourself.

What do you still need to make permanent lifestyle changes?
____

Do you need accountability?
____

Do you think you have an underlying medical condition?
____

Have you been giving this journey 100% of your effort?
____

Day 1: What did I eat today? What time(s) of the day did I eat?
____
____
____
____
____
____

MOVEMENT CHOICES: _______________________________________

Day 2: What did I eat today? What time(s) of the day did I eat?

____
____
____
____
____
____

MOVEMENT CHOICES: _______________________________

Day 3: What did I eat today? What time(s) of the day did I eat?

____
____
____
____
____
____

MOVEMENT CHOICES: _______________________________

Day 4 MOVEMENT CHOICES: ___________________________

Day 5 MOVEMENT CHOICES: ___________________________

We have worked on some serious lifestyle changes together, but you're on your own now. At any time you can go back and start the program over again. You can go back and do any week over again. And at any point you can reach out to me for a one on one consultation. Ask for help when you need it.

 Finally, don't make excuses as to why you can't do something, i.e. exercise, go to bed earlier, not eat the piece of bread etc.… I did that for too many years when it came to writing this book. That's why you have it in your hands now and not 5 years ago.

See you can blame me for your hold up on getting your body and health back on track. But now you have the book so you have no more excuses!

HOW TO CONTACT AND/OR WORK WITH AMIE:

So maybe you've discovered that you have a lot of health issues going on an would like to finally get your life back. Or maybe you are thinking a deeper look at your eating and lifestyle habits along with some serious accountability would serve you best. Then please keep reading more about Amie's services and how to get some personalized attention…

GETTING STARTED

Amie's priority is your health and continued wellness. She's in it for the long haul, but she can't do it for you. A better life is waiting for you, one filled with energy and new adventures, but it's up to YOU to make it happen!

So, the question is this: Are YOU ready to change your diet and lifestyle? Are YOU committed to improving your health and quality of life?

How to Contact Amie:

By Phone: 412.400.0828

By Email: amiehornaman@gmail.com

Visit Website: www.amiehornaman.com

Facebook: facebook.com/amiehornamannutrition

Amie Hornaman - owner, Amie Hornaman Nutrition and Functional Medicine

For over 20 years, Amie has helped people reclaim their health with Nutrition and Functional Medicine. Amie is a certified nutritionist with a Masters degree in Clinical Nutrition. She is also Erie's only Functional Medicine Practitioner, getting to the root cause of her client's health concerns, specializing in endocrinology. Because every client is unique, so is Amie's approach to their health.

Amie is honest and passionate about helping people reach their goals. She will tell you what you NEED to hear, NOT what you WANT to hear. She'll hold your hand and cheer you on, but she won't tell you that it's okay to eat bread and drink wine every day. Amie's passion to help is obvious in her accessibility for clients. A unique aspect of her program is 24/7 access to her as one of Amie's clients.

Amie's competitive/athletic background includes NPC and OCB fitness and figure competitions as well as RAW United and WABDL Powerlifting competitions, leading to work with collegiate and professional athletes in areas of nutrition and athletic performance.

Amie's extensive experience in clinical nutrition and functional medicine has made her a leader in the community in thyroid disorders, hormone imbalance and oncology nutrition. When asked what she does, Amie gives a simple answer of, "I fix people."

www.ingramcontent.com/pod-product-compliance
Lightning Source LLC
Chambersburg PA
CBHW080046260726
48658CB00007B/2771